NURTURING CHILDREN WITH DOWN SYNDROME:

A parent's guide to recognizing, coping and fostering growth.

Camilla Schoen

Table of contents

CHAPTER ONE:

Introduction

1.0. Overview of the book's goals.

Our main objective in conducting this thorough investigation is to offer a road map for parents, teachers, and other carers, promoting an awareness of Down syndrome from birth to adulthood. We start by going over the essentials, providing a precise description of Down syndrome and a thorough examination of its genetic causes.

Beyond comprehension, the book discusses the usefulness of early diagnosis and intervention, highlighting the critical importance of prompt detection and providing concrete methods to support a favorable developmental trajectory. Every chapter focuses on fostering important facets of a child's development, from emotional intelligence to effective communication.

Customized learning methods are in demand, with a focus on meeting the needs of each individual student and promoting inclusive teaching practices. The handbook broadens its scope to include children's overall health, covering both common health concerns and the encouragement of healthy lifestyles.

Social integration is promoted by having inclusive community conversations and building strong support networks. The book helps parents recognise and nurture their child's special talents by revealing their potential and examining creative expression and talent development.

Our book offers advice on career training, adolescent readiness, and the complexities of family support as kids grow into adulthood. We stress how critical it is to reinforce family bonds and provide parents and siblings with coping mechanisms.

Beyond the family unit, the manual promotes activism and community involvement. We hope to promote positive change by demonstrating interactions with organizations that help individuals with Down syndrome and emphasizing the role that families play in promoting inclusivity.

The book ends with a forward-looking look that celebrates encouragement and scientific progress. It ends with a recap of the most important lessons learned and an inspiring plea to embrace the incredible experience of raising children with Down syndrome. It asks readers to picture a world in which people with Down syndrome flourish.

1.1. Definition of Down syndrome

Trisomy 21, another name for Down syndrome, is a genetic disorder caused by an extra copy of chromosome 21. This extra genetic material has an impact on how the body and brain grow, which can cause difficulties with cognition and physical health. People with Down syndrome frequently have variable degrees of cognitive disability and may have distinguishing physical characteristics.

A chromosomal condition known as down syndrome is caused by an additional whole or partial copy of chromosome 21. This extra genetic material affects both physical and cognitive features, upsetting the usual path of development. People who have Down syndrome may have characteristic facial features, differing degrees of intellectual disability, and sometimes related health problems. The disorder is brought on by nondisjunction during cell division, which results in three copies of chromosome 21 rather than the normal two. The vast array of traits seen in people with Down syndrome is partly due to the intricacy of its genetic influence.

CHAPTER TWO:

Comprehension of down

syndrome

2.0. Deciphering the Genetic Tapestry: Genetics and the Origins of Down Syndrome.

The chromosomal abnormality known as Down syndrome is caused by a complicated interaction of genes. This disorder, commonly referred to as trisomy 21, develops when chromosome 21 is duplicated, changing the usual genetic makeup.

The phenomenon known as nondisjunction during cell division is the source of Down syndrome. This abnormality arises from improper chromosomal separation, which results in an extra copy of chromosome 21.

Approximately 95% of instances are caused by this trisomy 21 pattern. On the other hand, translocation and mosaicism explain a lower proportion of instances.

A combination of cells with varying chromosomal makeup is involved in mosaicism. Some cells in people with mosaic Down syndrome have the normal chromosomal layout, whereas other cells have the extra chromosome 21. On the other hand, translocation entails the attachment of a portion of chromosome 21 to a different chromosome. This kind could be hereditary or sporadic.

2.1. Common Aspects of the Down Syndrome Mind and Body: An Extensive Examination.

Due to an additional copy of chromosome 21, Down syndrome is characterized by a unique combination of physical and cognitive traits. Comprehending these shared attributes is vital in delivering sophisticated and encouraging healthcare.

Spatial Qualities:

The physical characteristics of people with Down syndrome are typically identifiable, including almond-shaped eyes, a flattened facial profile, and a smaller, flatter nose. Reduced muscle tone, a distinct hand and finger form, and a shorter stature are possible additional physical characteristics. Even though these characteristics add to the recognisable appearance, it's important to recognise the originality that falls within this range.

Mental Qualities:

There is a wide range of cognitive development in Down syndrome, from mild to substantial intellectual problems. Notwithstanding these differences, people with Down syndrome often exhibit noteworthy talents in emotional intelligence, interpersonal relationships, and social skills. To create a nurturing atmosphere that encourages personal development, it is essential to recognise and value certain cognitive traits.

Medical Considerations:

Beyond the obvious traits, people with Down syndrome may need to take certain health precautions. These can include a higher chance of thyroid issues, hearing and vision problems, and congenital cardiac anomalies. Ensuring comprehensive treatment and swiftly resolving possible difficulties require vigilant health management and early intervention.

CHAPTER THREE: Early diagnosis and intervention

3.0. The Value of Early Down Syndrome Detection.

Early identification of Down syndrome is like a lighthouse directing a child's life path, opening doors to specialized care and therapies. This proactive strategy, which is frequently implemented in the prenatal or infancy periods, is extremely beneficial to the individual as well as their carers.

1. Customising Interventions to Promote Optimal Growth:

Targeted therapies can be started quickly after early identification. Whether it be medical interventions, educational programmes, or therapeutic tactics, early detection of Down syndrome offers a critical window for applying individualized approaches. This customized help is essential for minimizing any problems and making the most of each person's developmental path.

2. Giving Families Access to Resources and Knowledge:

Families with children with Down syndrome can better handle the special challenges of raising their children when there is early discovery. By providing information about the disease, relevant health risks, and available support resources, it empowers parents and carers. Equipped with this knowledge, parents may make well-informed choices and cultivate a nurturing atmosphere for their child's development.

3. Promoting Emotional Health and Early Bonds:

Early identification of Down syndrome allows families to form close emotional relationships from the beginning. This early bond improves the child's emotional health as well as that of their carers, creating a loving and nurturing atmosphere that is essential for development as a whole.

4. Promoting Prompt Medical Interventions:

Early medical intervention may help with some Down syndrome-related health conditions. Early detection allows medical practitioners to take prompt action, enhancing overall quality of life and health outcomes, from treating congenital heart problems to managing hearing or vision issues.

To put it simply, early discovery of Down syndrome is crucial since it not only helps with diagnosis but also serves as a trigger for proactive, individualized care. It turns obstacles into opportunities, enabling people to reach their greatest potential and highlighting the significance of early support on the amazing journey of those who have Down syndrome.

3.1 Useful Down syndrome early intervention strategies techniques.

In order to maximize the potential of people with Down syndrome, promote development, and open doors to a happy life, early intervention is essential. Here, we explore useful and efficient methods that are intended to offer significant assistance in these critical initial phases.

1. Tailored Education Programmes:

Early intervention centers on creating individualized learning programmes that are specific to each child's strengths and problems. These plans take into account the child's preferences, cognitive profile, and developmental stage to make sure that interventions are both interesting and successful.

2. Therapy for Speech and Language:

Targeted speech and language therapy is frequently used in early intervention to improve communication abilities. In order to increase verbal and nonverbal communication, encourage expressive communication, and stimulate language development, speech therapists collaborate with families to present activities.

3. Development of Fine and Gross Motor Skills:

In early intervention, addressing the development of motor skills is essential. Using exercises that improve large and fine motor skills, occupational therapists help patients become more coordinated, balanced, and dexterous. Increased independence in day-to-day tasks is made possible by these therapies.

4. Developing Social Skills:

Training in social skills is included in early intervention to promote meaningful interactions. Children with Down syndrome can strengthen their social awareness, collaboration, and ability to form friendships through group activities, peer interactions, and planned play sessions.

5. Techniques for Integrating Sensations:

There may be variations in the way that many people with Down syndrome interpret sensory information. Early intervention uses sensory integration strategies to support people's ability to adjust and react appropriately to environmental cues. Activities that stimulate different senses to enhance sensory processing and self-regulation may be part of this.

6. Family-focused assistance:

Early intervention strategies take into account the significance of family involvement and aim to empower families. By giving parents and other carers the knowledge, tools, and continuous support they need, we can empower them to take an active role in their child's development and foster a cooperative, stimulating environment.

CHAPTER FOUR: Emotional Intelligence and Communication

4.0. Developing Resilience on an Emotional Level: A Manual for Increasing Emotional IQ in Children with Down Syndrome.

Starting the process of fostering emotional intelligence in kids with Down syndrome is a worthwhile endeavor that gives them the ability to handle the complexity of emotions with perseverance and grace. This is a thorough manual filled with helpful tips and compassion.

1. Creating an Emotional Bond:

Build a solid bond with your child to create a safe emotional foundation. Make bonding time a priority and partake in activities that elicit happy feelings. Developing a relationship based on trust is essential for emotional development.

2. Promoting Expression of Emotions:

Give your kids the freedom to use play, art, or language to communicate their feelings. Offer a variety of ways for people to express themselves, supporting the notion that all feelings are real. This facilitates the development of a sound emotional lexicon and helps with feeling comprehension and regulation.

3. Development of Social Skills:

Encourage social connections that lead to understanding and empathy. Take part in cooperative, sharing, and turn-taking activities to build interpersonal relationships and a feeling of community.

4. Accepting Emotional Learning:

Give your kids age-appropriate resources to help them learn about emotions. Utilize games, stories, or visual aids to assist kids in recognising and understanding various emotions. This helps them become more self-aware while also improving their emotional literacy.

5. Using relaxation and mindfulness techniques:

To assist your child in handling stress and navigating intense emotions, teach them basic mindfulness and relaxation techniques. Emotional control and wellbeing are enhanced by practices like guided imagery and deep breathing.

6. Developing Resilience in the Face of Adversity:

Encourage your youngster to view obstacles and failures as chances for personal development. As you assist children in addressing problems, stress the value of resilience and experience-based learning.

7. Creating a Happy Environment:

Establish a loving, caring atmosphere at home where people can freely express and celebrate their emotions. Highlight your child's qualities and strengths to help them feel confident and valuable.

By fostering emotional intelligence, we give children with Down syndrome the tools they need to not only recognise and control their emotions but also live resilient and satisfying lives. A brighter and more emotionally rich future is within reach with each step taken towards developing emotional intelligence.

4.1. Techniques for Improving Down syndrome Children's Communication Skills

Understanding and connection are based on effective communication. Strong communication skills are a life-changing experience that allows kids with Down syndrome to express themselves and engage in meaningful interactions with others. This is a manual full of useful tips to improve their communication skills.

1. Exposure to Early and Regular Communication:

Early and regular language introduction is recommended. Give your child a rich language experience, a diverse vocabulary, and verbal interactions all around them. A solid foundation for language growth and comprehension is laid by this exposure.

2. Making Use of Augmented Communication and Visual Aids:

To enhance verbal communication, include photos, visual aids, and other augmentative communication methods. By enhancing understanding and facilitating effective expression, this visual reinforcement closes the gap in communication.

3. Promotion of Speech Therapy:

Seek the assistance of speech therapists with experience in working with kids who have Down syndrome. Sessions of structured speech therapy can focus on certain issues and provide specialized techniques to improve speech articulation and clarity.

4. Play-Based Learning at Work:

Incorporate play activities that promote communication skills. In addition to making learning entertaining, games, role-playing, and interactive storytelling offer chances for language practice in a relaxed and interesting setting.

5. Creating Reliable Schedules:

Regular schedules that are both predictable and structured foster a positive environment for language development. Maintaining consistency helps kids feel secure, which makes it easier for them to anticipate and take part in linguistic conversations.

6. Facilitating Social Exchanges:

Promote social contacts among family members and peers. Playdates and group activities offer excellent chances to practice communication in a variety of settings, promoting social skills in addition to language development.

7. Honoring Minor Victories:

No matter how tiny, acknowledge and celebrate each communication milestone. A positive feedback loop is created, which increases self-assurance and encourages sustained effort.

8. Tailored Communication Strategies:

Work together with speech therapists and educators to create customized communication plans. Adapting tactics to each child's distinct communication style and preferences guarantees a customized and successful strategy.

By fostering their communication abilities, we enable kids with Down syndrome to express themselves, form relationships, and go confidently through life. Every effort made to improve their communication skills makes society more open-minded and communicative.

CHAPTER FIVE: Educational Approaches

5.0. Customising Educational Plans for Every Down Syndrome Student.

Developing an inclusive and successful educational experience requires an understanding of the distinct strengths and challenges that each child with Down syndrome faces. This is a how-to manual for creating personalized lesson plans that fulfill students' requirements and encourage a love of learning.

1. Entire Evaluations:

Start by carrying out comprehensive evaluations to ascertain the person's cognitive talents, preferred methods of learning, and particular areas that could need further assistance. This serves as the foundation for developing an individualized learning plan.

2. Personalized Learning Goals:

Create measurable learning goals that are appropriate for the child's skill level and learning speed. A favorable attitude towards education and drive are fostered by setting and achieving attainable goals.

3. Multimodal Methods of Education:

Use a range of sensory modalities in your instruction to meet the needs of different learning styles. Including visual aids, practical exercises, and audio stimulation increases student engagement and encourages a deeper comprehension of the material.

4. Adaptable Curriculum Changes:

Make necessary changes to the curriculum's pace, complexity, or content to meet the needs of each individual student. Because of this flexibility, every kid can advance at their own pace, resulting in a more individualized and encouraging learning environment.

5. Integration of Assistive Technology:

Examine how assistive technology that addresses certain learning needs can be integrated. Whether it's interactive applications, text-to-speech tools, or adaptive software, technology may be a strong ally in improving understanding and accessibility.

6. The cooperative team approach:

Encourage cooperation between parents, therapists, and educators to establish a strong support network. Frequent communication makes sure that everyone is taking the same approach, which creates a cohesive and reliable learning environment.

7. Emphasis of Social and Emotional Learning:

Give social and emotional learning materials top priority in the lesson plan. Prioritizing abilities like empathy, self-awareness, and effective communication enhances general wellbeing in addition to academic performance.

8. Frequent Progress Tracking:

Conduct assessments on a regular basis to track student development and modify lesson plans as necessary. This continuous assessment makes sure that the learning process is flexible and adaptable to the child's changing demands.

Through the process of creating individualized lesson plans, we set off on a revolutionary educational journey that honors and values every child's individuality. By doing this, we foster a passion for learning that goes well beyond the classroom and help students reach their full academic potential.

5.1. Cultivating Inclusive Education Strategies for Children with Down Syndrome

In the context of education, inclusive education is a potent catalyst for promoting diversity, acceptance, and equitable opportunity. Developing inclusive education practices for kids with Down syndrome involves more than just making accommodations; it also entails fostering an atmosphere where each student can succeed. This is a how-to for creating inclusive education plans that are both interesting and successful.

1. Tailored Education Programmes:

Set the stage for inclusivity by creating individualized lesson plans that address each child's particular needs and skills. Adapting teaching strategies guarantees that all students, including those with Down syndrome, get the assistance needed for a fulfilling educational experience.

2. Models of Collaborative Education:

Encourage cooperation amongst teachers, experts, and support personnel to build an inclusive team. Different points of view are included in lesson planning when using a collaborative teaching model, which makes it possible to take a more thorough approach to meeting student requirements.

3. Personalized Education:

To accommodate multiple learning styles in a single classroom, use differentiated instruction strategies. Every student is empowered by a variety of teaching strategies, resources, and evaluations, which promote an inclusive learning environment that values diversity.

4. Programmes for Peer Assistance and Mentoring:

Promote mentorship and peer support initiatives that foster constructive relationships between students. These kinds of programmes not only help students feel like they belong, but they also advance empathy, understanding, and support among one another in the classroom.

5. UDL stands for Universal Design for Learning.

Incorporate the concepts of Universal Design for Learning into your lesson planning to make sure that all students can access the instructional materials and methodologies. UDL promotes adaptability and flexibility by taking into account the various ways that students interact with and present their learning.

6. Practices for Sensory-Friendly Classrooms:

Incorporate components that address sensory needs to create a learning environment that is pleasant to all senses. These modifications guarantee a more welcoming and accommodating environment for every student, from taking into account lighting and seating configurations to offering sensory breaks.

7. Ongoing Professional Improvement:

To keep teachers up to date on the newest inclusive education strategies, provide them with continual professional development opportunities. Giving educators the resources and know-how they need to modify their approaches guarantees an inclusive, dynamic learning environment that is always changing.

8. All-inclusive After-School Activities:

By including kids with Down syndrome in extracurricular activities, you can promote inclusivity outside of the classroom. Offering possibilities for participation in activities, whether they be clubs, sports, or the arts, helps people feel like they belong and advance social integration.

Incorporating inclusive education practices fosters a diverse, accepting, and empathetic learning environment for students with Down syndrome as well as instills these values in the larger educational community. Adopting inclusion is a commitment to creating a learning environment where each and every student may succeed, not merely a goal in and of itself.

CHAPTER SIX: Health and Physical Wellbeing

6.0. Dealing with Physical Wellbeing: Techniques for Handling Common Health Concerns in People with Down Syndrome.

For people with Down syndrome, navigating the healthcare system calls for a proactive, comprehensive strategy. We can promote optimal well-being by treating common health conditions with a combination of education, preventative care, and supportive care. This is a how-to for handling typical health issues with tact and compassion.

1. Frequent Medical Examinations:

Establish a schedule for routine health checks in order to identify and address possible problems early on. Frequent examinations, such as thyroid screenings, vision and hearing tests, and cardiac evaluations, provide a proactive approach to managing prevalent health issues linked to Down syndrome.

2. Providers of Specialized Healthcare:

Work together with medical specialists who are skilled in handling the particular medical requirements of people with Down syndrome. Specialists in the field can provide information and treatments designed to address the unique health issues related to the illness.

3. Dental Care Priority:

Stress the importance of dental care as a component of total health management. Regular dental checkups and preventive care are essential for maintaining oral health since people with Down syndrome may be more susceptible to specific tooth problems.

4. Plans for Diet and Exercise:

Create individualized diet and fitness regimens to support general health and wellbeing. In addition to promoting physical health, a balanced diet and regular exercise also enhance mental and emotional wellbeing.

5. Support for Mental Health:

Acknowledge the significance of emotional and mental wellness. Provide channels for emotional support, such as support groups, counseling, or specialized therapies. A holistic approach benefits from treating mental health as a crucial aspect of general health.

6. Vaccine Adherence:

Follow advised immunization schedules to guard against diseases that can be avoided. Vaccinating people with Down syndrome on time is in line with preventative healthcare practices and protects their general health.

7. Active Involvement of the Carer:

Encourage carers to take an active role in managing healthcare. Giving carers the information they need to be proactive in promoting the health of their loved one—such as common health conditions, symptoms to look out for, and preventive measures—enables them to do so.

8. Being Ready for Emergencies:

Create disaster preparedness strategies that take any particular medical needs into account. A well-defined plan for handling medical crises guarantees a prompt and efficient reaction, enhancing the security and well-being of people with Down syndrome.

Through adopting a thorough and knowledgeable approach to common health issues, we not only address acute difficulties but also improve the long-term health and quality of life for people with Down syndrome. Ensuring that every individual receives the customized care and attention they require is made possible by incorporating healthcare within a comprehensive framework.

6.1. Promoting Healthy Lifestyles for People with Down Syndrome

Encouraging healthy lives for people with Down syndrome is a multifaceted endeavor that includes physical health, mental stability, and a dedication to general vitality. By cultivating constructive behaviors and offering customized assistance, we can enable people with Down syndrome to have happy, healthy lives. This is a manual for developing a well-being culture that is professional and involves real participation.

1. The Holistic Wellness Method:

Adopt a wellness philosophy that takes into account one's mental, emotional, and physical health. Understanding how these factors are related to one another paves the way for an all-encompassing and well-rounded approach to health.

2. Frequent Exercise:

Encourage frequent exercise that suits each person's tastes and abilities. Engaging in adaptive sports, leisure pursuits, or regular strolls are all excellent ways to keep active and improve mental and physical well-being.

3. Plans for Balanced Nutrition:

Create nutrient-dense, well-balanced meal plans based on each person's needs. Promote a varied and healthful diet that meets specific dietary needs, enhances general health, and helps maintain long-term energy levels.

4. Habits of Hydration:

Stress how crucial it is to maintain hydration. Drinking enough water is important for several body processes and promotes general health. Developing good hydration practices is an easy but important step towards wellbeing.

5. Tips for Good Sleep Hygiene:

Put proper sleep hygiene first because it's essential to leading a healthy lifestyle. The best slumber is facilitated by regular sleep schedules and the creation of a sleep-friendly atmosphere, which promotes both physical and mental health.

6. Practicing mindfulness and managing stress:

To improve emotional resilience, incorporate mindfulness exercises and stress reduction strategies. People who engage in mindful activities, relaxation techniques, and coping skills are better equipped to handle life's obstacles with poise and dignity.

7. Frequent Medical Examinations:

Suggest a proactive attitude to healthcare by arranging for routine examinations. Regular health examinations help with early detection and treatment of possible health problems, which is a component of preventative care.

8. bolstering Social Networks:

To improve emotional wellbeing, cultivate a network of supportive social relationships. Positive social interactions—whether through friendships, family ties, or community involvement—have a substantial positive impact on one's sense of overall satisfaction and belonging.

9. Lifelong Education and Development of Skills:

Encourage a culture that values skill development and lifelong learning. Cognitive well-being is enhanced by learning new abilities and partaking in mentally stimulating activities, which also enhance personal fulfillment.

Encouraging healthy living for people with Down syndrome not only addresses current health issues but also establishes the foundation for long-term vitality and fulfillment. This journey is a team effort that values and honors the distinct talents and strengths of each person, promoting a culture of well-being that goes well beyond the material world.

CHAPTER SEVEN: Social Integration

7.0. Promoting Down syndrome individuals' inclusion in the community.

The distinctive contributions of each and every person, including those with Down syndrome, must be acknowledged and celebrated in order to build a community that is truly inclusive. Through cultivating an atmosphere of tolerance, comprehension, and assistance, we may create an inclusive fabric that enhances the well-being of every individual in the community. This is a manual for promoting diversity in the community while maintaining professionalism and sincere involvement.

1. Programmes for Education and Awareness:

Launch educational and awareness campaigns in the neighborhood to debunk myths and advance knowledge of Down syndrome. Acquiring knowledge is the first step in promoting tolerance and celebrating differences.

2. Events and Activities That Are Allowed:

Plan occasions and pursuits that actively include people who have Down syndrome. Offering possibilities for involvement in events like sports, the arts, or community get-togethers promotes a feeling of integration and belonging.

3. Initiatives for Accessibility:

Put accessibility measures into practice to make community areas inclusive and hospitable to all. This goes beyond merely being physically accessible; it also involves offering information in different formats and taking changes that are sensory-friendly into account.

4. Peer groups and supportive networks:

Create peer groups and networks of support to help people with Down syndrome connect with one another. Initiatives led by the community that promote camaraderie, guidance, and mutual experiences enhance a feeling of being a part of the community.

5. Cooperation with Neighbourhood Companies:

Promote cooperation with nearby companies to generate inclusive job possibilities. Highlighting the varied skills and aptitudes of people with Down syndrome helps to create an inclusive work environment.

6. Honoring Successes and Milestones:

Celebrate in public the successes and life milestones of people with Down syndrome in the community. Acknowledging successes strengthens the community's resolve to accept diversity while also honoring the individual.

7. Strengthening Families and Carers:

Provide families and carers with resources and assistance. Families are made to feel supported and empowered in their journey by establishing a network of understanding and support throughout the community.

8. Initiatives for Inclusive Education:

Promote and back inclusive education programmes at your community's schools. From an early age, fostering conditions where all students, regardless of ability, study together fosters an inclusive culture.

9. Opportunities for Volunteering and Service:

Provide people with Down syndrome the chance to actively participate in the community by offering volunteer and service opportunities. Encouraging meaningful engagement fosters a sense of purpose and improves community inclusion overall.

10. Involve Influencers and Community Leaders:

Engage influential people and community leaders in the promotion of diversity. Through their advocacy, local attitudes, laws, and customs that support a more hospitable and inclusive atmosphere can be shaped.

In addition to improving the lives of those who have Down syndrome, our communities are strengthened when we proactively promote community inclusivity. Accepting variety turns into a common value that shapes the identity of the neighborhood and promotes empathy and social cohesion.

7.1. Establishing Robust Support Networks for Families with Down Syndrome.

Raising a child with Down syndrome presents unique challenges as well as pleasant experiences. Building strong support networks for families is essential to their resilience and overall wellbeing. This is a manual for creating professional and sincere support systems that empower and elevate families.

1. Peer Assistance Systems:

Encourage communication with families going through comparable situations. Peer support networks offer a forum for exchanging perspectives, obstacles, and achievements, cultivating a feeling of unity and comprehension among families.

2. Expert Guidance Services:

Provide professional counseling services with a focus on supporting families of individuals with Down syndrome. These programmes offer a private setting for coping mechanisms, emotional expression, and direction on how to handle different parts of the journey.

3. Workshops and Resources for Education:

Plan informative workshops that provide families with information about Down syndrome and pertinent caregiving techniques. Giving families access to educational materials helps them better handle the special challenges of raising a child with Down syndrome.

4. Services for Respite Care:

Incorporate services for respite care to give families periodic respites. It can be difficult to balance caregiving obligations, but respite care provides much-needed relief and improves the general well-being of the family.

5. Cooperative Planning for Healthcare:

Promote the use of therapists, educators, and medical professionals in collaborative healthcare planning. A well-coordinated strategy guarantees that the child with Down syndrome has all of his or her requirements met.

6. Programmes for Community Outreach:

Participate in community outreach initiatives to increase awareness and get support from the community. Increasing understanding throughout the community helps create a more accepting and stigma-free atmosphere for families.

7. Financial and Legal Advice:

Make legal and financial advice accessible, taking into account the special needs of families raising children with Down syndrome. Families often find it easier to manage the complex legal and financial issues when they receive professional assistance.

8. Platforms for Online Help:

Provide virtual venues where families can interact, exchange resources, and seek guidance by setting up online support systems. These networks of support are international in nature and transcend national borders.

9. Training in Advocacy:

Give families advocacy training so they can speak up for the needs and rights of their children. Through this programme, families can become more self-assured and actively involved in creating policies that benefit people with Down syndrome.

10. Together, we celebrate milestones:

Celebrate successes and landmarks as a group. No matter how tiny, celebrating and recognising accomplishments fosters a good and uplifted sense of camaraderie among families.

We strengthen the resilience of families with Down syndrome and build a community that is unified in compassion and understanding by creating a tapestry of robust support networks. Every support system designed serves as a pillar, sustaining the strength and well-being of families as they travel through life.

CHAPTER EIGHT: Creative Expression and Talent Development

8.0. Recognising and Developing Gifts in People with Down Syndrome.

Identifying and developing one's skills is a life-changing process that goes beyond self-imposed boundaries. This approach helps people with Down syndrome feel more fulfilled personally and enriches society in addition to showcasing their special talents. This is a how-to manual for recognising and nurturing talent with integrity and sincerity.

1. Comprehensive Talent Evaluation:

Perform a comprehensive talent assessment that extends beyond conventional metrics. Acknowledge and respect a wide variety of capabilities, from social and interpersonal skills to artistic and creative ability. The distinctive qualities of every person ought to be appreciated and cherished.

2. Customized Programmes for Skill Development:

Create skill-building programmes based on the interests and talents of each individual. By offering specialized training opportunities, people can explore their hobbies and improve their talents in a variety of disciplines, including music, art, athletics, and other activities.

3. Promoting Inquiry and Observation:

Establish a setting that inspires curiosity. To assist people in uncovering hidden skills, expose them to a variety of experiences and activities. Introducing someone to a wide variety of activities expands their horizons and piques their curiosity.

4. Mentoring and Counseling:

Provide mentorship programmes so that people can get advice from seasoned experts in the fields they are interested in. In addition to offering insightful advice, mentoring creates a relationship of support that accelerates both professional and personal development.

5. Methods of Inclusive Education:

Encourage the adoption of inclusive teaching strategies that incorporate talent development into the curriculum. Talents can flourish in an atmosphere that emphasizes individual capabilities and diversity in learning approaches.

6. Highlighting Accomplishments:

Provide venues for showcasing abilities and accomplishments. Acknowledgment from the public not only increases self-esteem but also helps alter society attitudes on the abilities of people with Down syndrome.

7. Tools and Adaptive Technologies:

Use methods and technologies that are adaptable to help build talent. Whether it's adapted sports equipment or assisted art gadgets, technology can be a key component in developing and revealing potential.

8. Building a Community of Support:

Create a welcoming environment that celebrates and supports a range of abilities.

People feel emboldened to express themselves in an inclusive setting, which promotes a sense of belonging and pride in their individual qualities.

9. Integration of Life Skills:

Combine the teaching of life skills with talent development. This method not only improves particular skills but also gives people useful skills that support their general independence and wellbeing.

10. Constant Appreciation and Feedback:

Throughout the talent development process, give constant praise and criticism. Positive reinforcement encourages people to keep discovering and honing their talents by reiterating the importance of effort and success.

By recognising and nurturing our skills, we set off on a shared path of empowerment and development. By accepting the range of skills that people with Down syndrome possess, we make a positive contribution to a culture that values human potential in all its manifestations.

8.1. Examining Creative and Artistic Channels for People with Down Syndrome

Exploring artistic and creative outlets is a dynamic and powerful path that provides opportunities for self-expression, personal development, and enrichment of society for those with Down syndrome. This is a manual for encouraging creativity while recognising the distinctive artistic abilities present in this dynamic community and doing it with professionalism and true participation.

1. Various Creative Forms:

Promote experimentation with a variety of artistic mediums, including performing arts like dance, theater, and music as well as visual arts like painting and drawing. Offering a variety of choices enables people to choose and develop their favorite creative activities.

2. Workshops and Classes for the Arts:

Lead creative programmes and workshops that are appropriate for a range of interests and ability levels. In addition to offering organized learning opportunities, these workshops foster inclusive environments where people feel free to express themselves.

3. Equipment and Supplies for Adaptive Art:

Make use of accessible art supplies and tools to improve accessibility. Adaptive components, such as ergonomic tools and specialized brushes, guarantee that artistic expression is inclusive and accommodating to a wide range of skills.

4. Projects of Collaborative Art:

Encourage cooperation by organizing group art projects. In addition to fostering a feeling of community, group projects inspire people to exchange concepts, methods, and sources of inspiration, weaving a creative tapestry together.

5. Programmes for Art Therapy:

Include art therapy programmes as part of a comprehensive strategy for mental health. Through artistic expression, people can share and process their feelings in a therapeutic way with the help of art therapy.

6. Opportunities for Exhibitions:

Provide people with the chance to exhibit their artistic works. In addition to showcasing their talents, putting on exhibitions or performances helps to promote inclusivity and shift attitudes in the larger community.

7. Technology Integration:

Use technology to further your artistic research. Whether it's virtual reality experiences, software for composing music, or digital art platforms, technology can be a potent tool that helps people connect with and enhance their creative expression.

8. Programmes for Adaptive Dance and Movement:

Introduce programmes for adaptive dance and movement to investigate physicality as a medium for creative expression. These programmes are inclusive and offer a safe space for people of all abilities to express themselves and connect with their bodies.

9. Promoting Writing and Storytelling:

Encourage writing and storytelling as extra creative outlets. Encouraging people to share their tales, whether via digital narratives, poetry, or conventional storytelling, promotes a sense of agency and voice.

10. Honoring Creative Accomplishments:

Honor creative successes and landmarks. In addition to giving people with Down syndrome more self-assurance, acknowledging and appreciating their achievements and inventiveness also helps to foster a culture that values and accepts a variety of abilities.

Through exploring artistic and creative avenues, we set out on a path of self-discovery and empowerment. We support and celebrate the artistic expressions of people with Down syndrome, fostering a more diverse and culturally enriched community that values the beauty found in each individual's singular viewpoint.

CHAPTER NINE: Moving Up to Childhood

9.0. Preparing for Adolescence and Beyond with Down Syndrome.

When people with Down syndrome enter adolescence and beyond, it is a time of personal development, self-exploration, and opportunity. A dedication to promoting independence, careful planning, and support are necessary in order to be ready for this trip. Here's a how-to for handling these changes with poise and sincere interest, making sure the way forward supports and welcomes each person's developing potential.

1. Tailored Transition Strategies:

Create individualized transition plans that take into account each person's particular goals, interests, and strengths. These plans target academic, vocational, and life skills development and act as road maps for navigating adolescence and beyond.

2. Career & Vocational Exploration:

Start vocational and career exploration programmes to assist people in identifying their areas of interest and possible career pathways. Promoting early exposure to a variety of professions lays the groundwork for making well-informed judgements regarding one's future goals.

3. Training in Life Skills:

Include instruction on life skills into everyday activities. Possessing practical life skills improves independence and boosts general well-being. These abilities range from budgeting and time management to maintaining personal hygiene.

4. Development of Social Skills:

Give developing social skills a lot of attention. Participating in social contact, collaboration, and relationship-building activities gives people the skills necessary to make meaningful relationships in both their personal and professional life.

5. Ongoing Assistance with Education:

Continue to support education in a way that respects each student's unique interests and learning style. Developing a passion of learning is still an important part of becoming ready, whether through conventional academic routes or non-traditional educational methods.

6. Programmes for Independent Living:

Examine independent living programmes that provide safe spaces for people with Down syndrome to practice and develop everyday living skills. These initiatives offer a step towards increased independence.

7. Promotion of Self-Advocacy:

Encourage people to take up self-advocacy. To help children feel like they have agency and self-determination, encourage them to express their preferences, set goals, and actively engage in decision-making processes.

8. Support for Mental and Emotional Health:

Acknowledge how crucial it is to have mental and emotional support during this change. Access to tools, coping mechanisms, and counseling helps people maintain their mental health and resilience while navigating the difficulties of adolescence and adulthood.

9. Initiatives for Social Inclusion:

Encourage community-wide activities for social inclusion. Activities that promote involvement in clubs, social gatherings, and neighborhood associations help people feel connected and at home outside of their families and schools.

10. Cooperative Transition Arrangements:

Encourage cooperation amongst support staff, educators, and carers when it comes to transition planning. A cohesive strategy guarantees that the person gets all-encompassing assistance in all areas of their changing life.

Getting ready for adolescence and beyond is a group effort that honors and acknowledges the changing abilities of people with Down syndrome. We enable them to embrace the new chapters of their individual journey and traverse this exciting phase with confidence and optimism by offering them individualized assistance, encouragement, and growth possibilities.

9.1. Professional and Trade Education for People with Down Syndrome**

For people with Down syndrome, starting a professional and vocational training programme is a critical step towards their independence, self-determination, and meaningful contribution to society. Personalized support, skill development, and a dedication to creating inclusive workplaces are all part of this revolutionary process. This is a how-to guide for career and vocational training that unlocks prospects for meaningful and purposeful futures with professionalism and true participation.

1. Tailored Career Evaluations:

Individualized career assessments that pinpoint interests, strengths, and possible career pathways should be used to kick off the process. Personalized training and career planning are built on an understanding of each person's distinct abilities.

2. Programmes for Developing Skills:

Develop skill development programmes that are in line with the needs of prospective careers as well as the aspirations of the participants. A variety of talents, including soft skills and technical competences essential for success in the workplace, should be covered in these programmes.

3. Careers and Relevant Experiences:

Encourage practical experiences and internships to give people a direct look at various job contexts. Practical experiences improve confidence and a feeling of professional identity in addition to improving skill mastery.

4. Career Guidance and Mentoring:

Implement mentorship and job coaching programmes to offer continuous advice and assistance in the workplace. In addition to helping people navigate the complexities of particular occupations and professional situations, a supportive mentoring promotes a feeling of belonging.

5. Easily accessible workplaces:

Promote and design inclusive workplaces that can accommodate a range of abilities. An inclusive work environment, assistive technology, and physical accommodations all help to create a supportive environment for people with Down syndrome.

6. Partnerships for Cooperation with Employers:

Form cooperative alliances with companies that are dedicated to inclusion and diversity. Involving companies in the training process promotes a culture of acceptance and support while also ensuring congruence with industry needs.

7. Opportunities for Ongoing Education:

As people advance in their jobs, encourage them to seek more education and training to foster a culture of lifelong learning. This dedication to continuous improvement fosters career advancement and flexibility.

8. Professional Development and Networking:

Promote networking and involvement in events for professional growth. People can increase their professional networks and keep up with industry trends by participating in industry networks and going to pertinent events.

9. Initiatives for Training Entrepreneurs:

Examine programmes offering entrepreneurship training to people who want to launch their own companies. Giving people the abilities and know-how to start their own business encourages self-reliance and autonomy in their professional endeavors.

10. Honoring Professional Milestones:

Celebrate professional accomplishments and turning points as people advance in their careers. Acknowledging successes not only raises spirits but also helps to alter public attitudes on the skills of people with Down syndrome in the workforce.

Every move made in the field of career and vocational training contributes to the creation of a workforce that is more varied and inclusive. Through individualized assistance, skill development, and cooperative partnerships, we open doors for people with Down syndrome to pursue rewarding careers, make significant contributions to their communities, and inspire a paradigm shift in societal attitudes regarding workplace inclusion.

CHAPTER TEN: Family Dynamics and Support

10.0. Fortifying Links with a Down Syndrome Child.

Raising a kid with Down syndrome is a unique adventure that involves both obstacles and rewards that strengthen family ties. Fostering compassion, honest communication, and a shared dedication to the welfare of each family member are all necessary to strengthen these bonds. This is a manual for developing solid family relationships with professionalism and sincere interest.

1. Honest and transparent communication:

Provide the groundwork for frank and open communication inside the family. A family atmosphere where everyone feels heard and encouraged is created by promoting conversation about feelings, difficulties, and victories.

2. All-Inclusive Family Events:

Include inclusive family activities that are tailored to each member's interests and capabilities, including the child who has Down syndrome. Shared experiences, such as hobbies and outings, foster a sense of joy and community.

3. Knowledge and Consciousness:

Encourage your family members to learn more about Down syndrome. Comprehending the ailment, its difficulties, and its distinct advantages cultivates compassion, endurance, and a group determination to surmount roadblocks jointly.

4. Joint Accountabilities:

Assign duties to family members so that caring obligations are divided. This cooperative method lessens the workload while reinforcing the notion that each family member is vital to the overall health of the family.

5. Systems of Emotional Support:

Create systems of emotional support for each other in the family. Recognise that every family member may have unique emotional requirements, and that building a mutually supportive environment helps to bolster resilience and cohesion.

6. Honoring Successes, Great and Small:

Celebrate each family member's accomplishments, no matter how minor. Recognising and celebrating accomplishments strengthens the value of shared joys and creates a good and upbeat family culture.

7. Participation in a Child's Development:

Include family members in the child's development, including updates on their health, therapy sessions, and academic achievements. This involvement fosters a sense of shared responsibility as well as a collaborative approach to the child's growth.

8. The Creation of Family Customs:

Establish and preserve family customs that unite the whole family. Whether they are associated with holidays, unique events, or daily activities, these customs support a feeling of consistency, continuity, and shared history.

9. Fostering Sibling Bonds:

By promoting communication and understanding between siblings, you can cultivate excellent sibling relationships. Sibling relationships are strengthened when shared activities, conversations, and support are given, forming a network of support for the child with Down syndrome.

10. Expert Assistance and Guidance:

When necessary, seek out professional counseling and support. Managing the difficulties of parenting a kid with Down syndrome can be difficult, but expert advice can offer coping mechanisms, improve family dynamics, and create a happy atmosphere.

In the context of Down syndrome, strengthening family bonds is a lifelong process of love, comprehension, and mutual development. Families may create a strong foundation that welcomes the difficulties and rewards of the amazing journey they go on together by encouraging open communication, showing support for one another, and appreciating the individuality of every family member.

10.1. Coping Strategies for Parents and Siblings of People with Down Syndrome:

Raising a child with Down syndrome is a special and fulfilling adventure that has its own set of obstacles and victories. Developing coping mechanisms is crucial for parents and siblings to travel this unique route together and with resilience. Here's how to manage both professionalism and sincere involvement while creating a nurturing atmosphere for parents and siblings.

1. Open Lines of Communication:

Create channels of open communication inside the family. Fostering candid conversations about feelings, worries, and successes makes room for understanding and support between people.

2. Welcoming Emotional Communication:

Recognise and accept a variety of feelings. In order to cope, a person must acknowledge that both joys and obstacles are essential components of the journey and allow oneself to feel and express emotions without restriction.

3. Creating a Network of Support:

Establish a network of friends, family, and professionals to help you. Talking about your experiences and thoughts with people who are aware of the particular difficulties you face can offer insightful viewpoints and emotional support.

4. Tips for Self-Care:

Make self-care routines a priority for both parents and siblings. Retaining emotional resilience and well-being requires making time for personal interests, hobbies, and downtime.

5. Empowerment and Education:

Spend time educating others about Down syndrome so that parents and siblings can make informed decisions. Acquiring knowledge about the illness helps debunk misconceptions, promotes acceptance, and provides the family with resources to deal with obstacles.

6. Resources for Therapy:

Investigate healing channels for expressing your emotions. These resources, which might include family or individual counseling, offer a secure setting for processing feelings, developing coping mechanisms, and fortifying family ties.

7. Participation of Siblings in Care:

Siblings should assist in providing care. In addition to improving the child's wellbeing, encouraging a sense of shared responsibility also helps to fortify the sibling bond through cooperative efforts.

8. Establishing Reasonable Expectations:

Celebrate little accomplishments and have reasonable expectations. Acknowledging and valuing any kind of progress—no matter how small—helps foster optimism and eases the burden on parents and siblings.

9. Building Sibling Relationships:

Sibling relationships can be strengthened by promoting quality time and common interests. Nurturing the special role that siblings play in each other's lives goes a long way towards building a solid and encouraging family dynamic.

10. Empowerment and Advocacy:

Promote parental and sibling empowerment and advocacy. Engaging in advocacy campaigns, support groups, and community participation gives the family the ability to make a good difference and increase awareness.

Parents' and siblings' coping strategies combine self-care, education, and emotional support.

Families may manage the challenges of raising a child with Down syndrome with strength and unity by building a culture of understanding, resilience, and shared responsibility. This allows families to turn obstacles into opportunities for connection and progress.

CHAPTER ELEVEN:

Community

11.0. Encouraging Families to Foster Inclusivity through the Cultivation of Inclusive Homes.

In order to create a society that honors and embraces diversity, inclusive families are essential. Creating an inclusive atmosphere is a celebration of individual skills and viewpoints as well as a commitment for families that have members with Down syndrome. Here's how to empower families to promote diversity inside the family by supporting them with professionalism and sincere participation.

1. Open Discussions Regarding Diversity:

Start frank discussions about diversity in the family. Talk on how each family member is special, highlighting the importance of individuality and creating a welcoming atmosphere.

2. Honor personal accomplishments:

Celebrate each family member's accomplishments on an individual basis and give them due recognition. The belief that every family member, regardless of skill, contributes to the prosperity of the group as a whole is reinforced by this practice.

3. Equitable Accountabilities and Inputs:

Encourage a sense of shared accountability and input. Recognise that everyone has something important to contribute, even those who have Down syndrome, whether it be to everyday tasks or decision-making.

4. All-Inclusive Family Events:

Include activities that are inclusive of all family members and take into account their individual interests and skills. Creating opportunities for shared experiences, such as game evenings and outings, improves familial relationships and promotes diversity.

5. Information on Down syndrome:

Encourage family education about Down syndrome. Comprehending the illness, its obstacles, and its distinct advantages cultivates compassion and establishes a basis for reassuring and knowledgeable familial relationships.

6. Promote Sibling Relationships:

Promote close relationships between siblings and stress the value of helping one another. In addition to being essential in promoting inclusivity, siblings also help to create a strong support system inside the family.

7. Take Part in Events Promoting Community Inclusion:

Engage in community inclusion events with vigor. Engaging the family in extracurricular inclusiveness-promoting activities helps to shift cultural beliefs while also fostering a feeling of belonging.

8. Easily accessible living spaces:

Establish accessible living spaces that meet a range of demands. A welcoming family environment is facilitated by offering assistive technologies, ensuring physical accessibility, and making modifications that promote inclusivity.

9. Encourage empowerment and advocacy:

Give family members the tools they need to promote inclusivity. Fostering proactive involvement in advocacy campaigns and community outreach reaffirms the family's dedication to advancing diversity in a wider context.

10. Foster an Environment of Respect:

Establish a respectful environment where the thoughts, feelings, and opinions of each family member are respected. Respect builds the foundation for candid dialogue and mutual understanding within the family.

Fostering a culture of tolerance within families is a path of mutual understanding, diversity celebration, and shared values. Families that celebrate the individual qualities of each member foster harmony inside the family as well as a larger movement in society towards tolerance and respect for diversity.

11.1. Successful Communication with Groups Assisting People with Down Syndrome

Working with groups that assist people with Down syndrome is a cooperative step towards empowerment, advocacy, and building an inclusive community. Here's guidance for anyone involved in these interactions—parents, carers, advocates—on how to handle them professionally and with genuine interest so that you may all work towards the common goal of improving the lives of people with Down syndrome.

1. Investigate and comprehend the company:

Do your homework to learn about the organization's goals, core principles, and particular support services before contacting them. The basis for meaningful and knowledgeable interactions is this knowledge.

2. Create Channels of Open Communication:

Establish open lines of communication with the company. Encouraging open and frequent communication, whether via phone, email, or in-person meetings, improves the partnership and guarantees goal alignment.

3. Attend workshops and events:

Engage in active participation in the workshops and events that the organization hosts. This participation not only offers insightful information and helpful resources, but it also shows that you are dedicated to lifelong learning and teamwork.

4. Talk About Your Own Experiences and Learnings:

Give the organization a glimpse into your personal experiences and observations. Giving firsthand accounts enhances the organization's approach to help by deepening understanding of the difficulties faced by people with Down syndrome and their families.

5. Work together on advocacy projects:

Investigate working together on advocacy projects. The impact of the group's advocacy for legislative changes, public awareness campaigns, and inclusive communities is increased when people work together to help people with Down syndrome.

6. Look for Resources and Guidance:

Don't be afraid to ask the organization for advice and resources. Making use of the organization's knowledge base to obtain information on therapies, educational materials, or coping mechanisms improves your capacity to offer the best possible help.

7. Provide Your Knowledge and Experience:

Think about donating your knowledge and abilities to the company. Whether through volunteer labor, event planning, or specialized expertise, your distinct perspective and talents can be invaluable assets in furthering the organization's objective.

8. Work Together on Educational Projects:

Work together on educational projects that advance knowledge and comprehension of Down syndrome. Collaborating in educational initiatives such as workshops, seminars, or informational campaigns helps dispel myths and promote a society with greater knowledge.

9. Give constructive criticism:

When required, offer constructive criticism. In order to better meet the needs of people with Down syndrome and their families, the organization's programmes and services are shaped by your involvement as a parent, carer, or advocate.

10. Together, let's celebrate accomplishments:

Together, celebrate successes and major anniversaries. Acknowledging and celebrating victories together not only improves your working relationship but also fosters a supportive and inspiring work atmosphere.

Engaging with Down syndrome support organizations requires more than just transactional interactions; it's a collaborative endeavor. Through encouraging candid dialogue, reciprocal education, and collective advocacy, you add to a support system that empowers people with Down syndrome and promotes good change more broadly.

CHAPTER TWELVE: Future Outlook and Innovations

11.0. Encouragement and Research Advancement:

Encouraging people and research advances can be transformative in the quest for development and good change for people with Down syndrome. Here's a handbook for anyone working in the field of caregiving, advocacy, or research to help you navigate this changing environment with professionalism and sincere involvement and create an endless future.

1. Honour Research Milestones:

Celebrate and recognise achievements in the field of down syndrome research.

Acknowledging accomplishments, whether they be novel therapy approaches or advances in the study of genetic variables, encourages optimism and drive throughout the community.

2. Encourage Research Projects:

Encourage and assist current research projects. Your engagement can be in clinical trials, raising money, creating awareness, or any other way that helps expand scientific understanding and improve the lives of people with Down syndrome.

3. Keep Up with Research Results:

Keep up with the most recent study discoveries. Continually interact with credible papers, sources, and research updates to increase your comprehension of the changing field of Down syndrome research.

4. Promote Funding for Research:

Encourage more financing for research. Your voice can play a significant role in increasing public awareness of the value of funding research on Down syndrome, which can ultimately hasten scientific discoveries and progress.

5. Take Part in Cooperative Research:

Examine possibilities for joint research projects. Fostering collaborative initiatives improves the interdisciplinary aspect of research on Down syndrome and promotes a holistic approach, regardless of whether one is a researcher, carer, or advocate.

6. Encourage the use of inclusive research methods.

Encourage inclusive research methods that give the perspectives and experiences of people with Down syndrome and their families first priority.

Research that is inclusive makes ensuring that different viewpoints are included in the creation of therapies and support systems that work better.

7. Motivate Future Researchers:

Mentor and encourage upcoming new researchers in the subject. Encouraging the next generation of researchers ensures that the pursuit of knowledge and innovation continues, and that the goal of bettering the lives of people with Down syndrome remains a constant.

8. Tell Your Own Tales:

Tell personal tales that illustrate the significance of scientific discoveries. Personal stories give scientific advancement a human face, igniting optimism and demonstrating the real advantages of research for people and families.

9. Promote the Use of Ethical Research Procedures:

Promote moral research procedures that put the dignity and well-being of people with Down syndrome first. Maintaining ethical norms in research enhances the legitimacy and reliability of scientific discoveries.

10. Establish a Positive Culture:

Encourage a positive and upbeat atmosphere among people with Down syndrome. Your support and encouragement help foster a mindset that values possibilities, resiliency, and a common dedication to a future in which people with Down syndrome are successful.

Research developments and encouragement work together to create a future full of possibilities and promise for people with Down syndrome. Participating actively in the research landscape, supporting moral behavior, and cultivating an optimistic culture make you an essential component of the transformative process leading to a more promising and inclusive future.

12.1. Imagining a Helpful Future for People with Down Syndrome:

Imagining a future for individuals with Down syndrome is an opportunity to create a tapestry of compassion, inclusivity, and limitless possibilities on the canvas of our collective ambitions. Together, as worldwide community members, carers, and advocates, let's set out to envisage a helpful future that recognises each person with Down syndrome for their individual talents and potential.

1. Inclusive Learning Environments:

Imagine a time when inclusive educational environments are a given. According to this vision, learning settings and institutions fluidly adjust to accommodate a wide range of learning styles, guaranteeing that every person—including those with Down syndrome—receives a customised and powerful education.

2. The Holistic Approach to Healthcare:

Imagine a holistic approach being embraced by the healthcare system. In this future, people with Down syndrome receive comprehensive, individualized treatment that prioritizes their mental, emotional, and general well-being in addition to their physical demands.

3. Integrated Vibrant Community:

Imagine living in a neighborhood where diversity is ingrained in the culture. In this picture, people with Down syndrome engage fully in communal life, making friends and sharing their special skills. Respect for one another and a sense of belonging are fostered in a community that values difference.

4. Helpful Career Prospects:

Imagine a workplace that is inclusive of people with Down syndrome. Workplaces in the future will foster diversity and offer fulfilling employment options. People with Down syndrome are empowered to follow their passions and actively participate in a variety of sectors.

5. Innovative Research Advancements:

Imagine new discoveries regarding Down syndrome that expand on existing possibilities. According to this theory, continuous scientific progress opens up new treatments, approaches, and insights. Research becomes a ray of hope, bringing cutting-edge fixes and improving the general quality of life for people with Down syndrome.

6. Universal Access to Technology:

Imagine a time when everyone has access to technology. According to this vision, technological advancements put inclusion first by providing adaptive solutions that enable people with Down syndrome to interact with and take use of the digital world, promoting their freedom and connectedness.

7. Empowerment thru Protest:

Imagine a society in which advocacy knows no bounds. In this future, campaigns for social justice raise public awareness, eradicate stigma, and promote understanding among the populace. The voices of people who have Down syndrome and those who support them grow into potent forces for good.

8. Honoring Special Talents:

Imagine living in a society that values each person's distinct abilities. This vision honors and celebrates artistic, creative, and individual achievements, fostering a community that supports and recognises the range of abilities among people with Down syndrome.

9. Strengthening family networks:

Imagine strong, nurturing familial networks. Families of people with Down syndrome will have access to resources, information, and a robust support network in the future, enabling them to create an atmosphere in which each member of the family can flourish.

10. An Equitable Opportunity World:

See a society in which everyone has equal access to opportunity. In this vision, people with Down syndrome go through a world where social norms do not restrict their ability to pursue their dreams. A world where everyone has equal opportunity is evidence of each person's intrinsic value and potential.

Let compassion, inclusivity, and a shared commitment to bringing to reality a world where each person is valued for the unique gifts they bring to humanity inspire us as we collectively paint this picture of a helpful future for people with Down syndrome.

CHAPTER THIRTEEN:

Conclusion

13.0. Crucial Lessons Learned from Raising Children with Down Syndrome.

As we come to the end of this fascinating investigation into raising children with Down syndrome, let's condense the complexity of our experience into a few important lessons that capture the spirit of empowerment, empathy, and understanding:

1. Accepting Diversities:

The embrace of difference is essential to our comprehension. Every child with Down syndrome has its individual set of abilities, perspectives, and skills. Accepting this diversity makes life richer for all of us and opens the door to a society where everyone is treated equally.

2. Early Identification and Reaction:

One cannot stress the importance of early detection and intervention. Early detection and focused treatments create the ideal environment for growth, giving kids with Down syndrome the assistance they require to succeed in a variety of spheres of life.

3. Developing Intelligence in Emotions:

The development of emotional intelligence becomes a fundamental component. Supporting the growth of emotional intelligence, resilience, and social skills in children with Down syndrome not only improves their overall wellbeing but also helps them form deep and meaningful relationships.

4. Tailored Learning Programmes:

The personalisation of lesson plans is highly beneficial. Children with Down syndrome can interact with learning in a way that best fits their specific learning styles when educational techniques are customized to meet their requirements. This encourages a love of learning.

5. Educational Inclusivity:

Strategies for inclusive education provide access to a world of opportunities. Establishing learning environments where children with Down syndrome attend school alongside their peers fosters understanding, dismantles barriers, and equips them to engage fully in a variety of social contexts.

6. Wholesome Health and Welfare:

Managing common health problems and promoting healthy lifestyles are multifaceted endeavors. Setting physical health, mental health, and general lifestyle choices as top priorities guarantees a holistic approach to nurturing the whole person.

7. Support networks and social integration:

A supportive atmosphere is built on the foundations of fostering community inclusivity and establishing robust support networks. Children with Down syndrome benefit from having strong support networks and making relationships within the community for a well-rounded growth.

8. Opening Up the Creative Process:

Finding and honing one's skills as well as exploring artistic and creative outlets open doors for self-expression. Unlocking one's creative potential promotes happiness, accomplishment, and a greater awareness of one's own strengths.

9. Getting Ready for Adulthood:

Strategic planning is necessary to prepare for adolescence and beyond as we look to the future. In addition to family dynamics and continuous support, career and vocational training helps prepare people with Down syndrome for a happy adult life.

10. Views for the Future and Advocacy:

We are steadfast in our commitment to advocating for and seeing a positive future. We contribute to a future in which people with Down syndrome are acknowledged, respected, and empowered by actively engaging in community involvement, interacting with organizations, and funding scientific developments.

These lessons serve as a road map for our joint investigation, showing the way ahead. May they provide motivation to keep working towards helping each child with Down syndrome reach their full potential and create a society that values and celebrates their special contributions.

13.1. Setting Out on the Unusual Adventure: A Down Syndrome Motivational Journey.

Life is an amazing journey, and for those who are impacted by Down syndrome, it becomes a singular and unforgettable experience. Let us take courage from the remarkable parts of this adventure and welcome the unorthodox with a positive and resilient attitude.

1. Accepting Individuality:

The embrace of individuality is at the core of the unusual adventure. Each person with Down syndrome has unique abilities, perspectives, and qualities to offer. It's a call to rejoice in the richness that diversity brings to life's fabric.

2. Adaptability at Every Turn:

We use resilience as our compass during this journey. People who have Down syndrome are incredibly strong, resilient, and determined. Every stride, no matter how big or tiny, bears witness to the unwavering spirit that permeates this incredible adventure.

3. Revealing Latent Skills:

Treasures of hidden talents are waiting to be discovered in this fascinating quest. Recognising and developing the special talents that people with Down syndrome bring to the surface can lead to a world of excitement and discovery, ranging from artistic expressions to surprising talents.

4. Creating Powerful Bonds:

Making relationships is the goal of the journey; it is not a lonely one. Communities, friends, and families unite in mutual understanding and support. Every relationship that is established is significant, highlighting the value of life experiences shared and group development.

5. Honoring Successes, Great and Small:**

Every accomplishment on this quest is worth celebrating. Whether the goal is to acquire a new ability, accomplish a goal, or just find happiness in small triumphs every day, the path is filled with moments of success that should be celebrated and acknowledged.

6. An Educational Journey:

Think of the odd journey as an ongoing educational experience. It teaches empathy, fortitude, and the value of having a variety of viewpoints. It dispels myths, opens doors, and encourages a lifelong quest for self-awareness.

7. Advocacy as a Light to Follow:

On this special route, advocacy takes on the role of a compass. Our efforts to promote inclusivity, dispel prejudices, and elevate voices pave the way for a time when people appreciate and even rejoice in the unexpected trip.

8. Crafting a Story that Empowers:

The trip is a story waiting to be written, a powerful tale of development, achievements, and the beauty that can be found at every turn. We can reshape cultural beliefs and provide a path towards a more compassionate and inclusive world by crafting a positive story.

9. Accepting Difficulties as Chances:

Obstacles are not barriers to advancement; rather, they present possibilities. Every obstacle becomes an opportunity to demonstrate adaptation, tenacity, and the amazing ability to transform setbacks into steps towards a better future.

10. Motivating Hope for the Future:

Upon starting this extraordinary journey, we transform into rays of hope. We encourage optimism for future generations as well as for ourselves by welcoming the trip with open minds and hearts—a world in which people with Down syndrome are respected, included, and honored.

Motivated by the tremendous possibilities this unexpected experience contains, let's embrace it with open arms. Let the celebration of accomplishments be our constant companion on this incredible voyage, let uniqueness serve as our compass, and let resilience be our guide through every twist and turn.